I0416575

Heart Disease (Heart Attack)

Guide To A Healthy Heart

By

Brian A. Godfrey

TABLE OF CONTENTS

INTRODUCTION

Welcome to the empowering realm of "Heart Disease (Heart Attack): Guide to a Healthy Heart." The rich tapestry that is our life is woven with the intricate role that our hearts play, and they are pulsating with the rhythm of vitality. Your passport to understanding, avoiding, and fostering a heart that beats with resilience and energy is this complete guide, which is your passport to all of these things.

We will shed light on the intricacies that distinguish a heart attack from the symphony of life as we embark on this instructive trip. As we do so, we will uncover the complexities of heart illness.

A heart that lives in spite of the challenges of modern existence is illuminated by this guide, which is more than just a road map; it is a lighthouse that illuminates the path to that heart.

Every single chapter serves as a gateway into the realm of cardiovascular health, providing you with actionable advice and solutions that are supported by scientific research, thereby enabling you to take charge of your cardiovascular destiny. The information contained in these pages is a treasure trove of knowledge that is geared at cultivating a healthy and long-lasting heart. It includes heart-friendly exercises as well as heart-boosting foods.

Come along with us as we make our way through the pages of prevention, identifying the signs and taking the steps that will strengthen your heart against the winds of possible difficulties. The book "Heart Disease (Heart Attack): Guide to a Healthy Heart" is more than simply a book; it is your reliable travel companion on the path to a life that is full of vitality and heart health. With an open heart and a willingness to embrace the information that can change fear into empowerment and uncertainty into resilience, you should go on this journey. Your heart's health is a key melody, and this book is the conductor that teaches you to compose a symphony of a healthy, lively heart.

CHAPTER ONE

The Remarkable Heart

Circulatory system, also known as the cardiovascular system, is made of the heart and an astonishing number of arteries, veins, and capillaries that carry blood to every extremity of your body. There is a lot to talk here, so let's start by having a careful look at the heart. We have a tendency to romanticize the heart, and in the past, we have even assigned it as a center of cognition and emotion. We now know that this is not accurate, as the brain is where all of that activity takes place, while the heart, which resides within the medial cavity of the thorax known as the mediastinum, serves just as a pump. But this doesn't make it any less spectacular, as we shall discover. The first thing we must bring out is that the heart participates in two circuits. Blood enters the right side of the heart and is directed to the lungs where it becomes oxygenated. When the oxygen we breathe in from the air around us diffuses through the lungs and into the circulation to bind to hemoglobin, then this returns to the left side of the heart to complete the pulmonary circuit. Then, the oxygenated blood exits the left side of the heart and is distributed throughout the body to give oxygen and nutrients to all the numerous tissues that need oxygen to accomplish cellular respiration.

It unloads all that oxygen and ultimately makes it back to the right side of the heart, thus completing the systemic circuit. So, we have two circuits and two reception chambers in the heart where these cycles terminate, those being the right atrium and left atrium. Along with them, there are two primary pumping chambers, those being the right ventricle and left ventricle. The heart is covered by something called the pericardium, which is formed of strong connective tissue that protects the heart and maintains its position.

The two walls of the pericardium are the fibrous pericardium and the serous pericardium, the latter of which also contains two layers, the parietal layer and the visceral layer, also known as the epicardium.

The epicardium is considered the outermost layer of the heart wall, the others being the myocardium and endocardium.
The myocardium makes up most of the heart, and it is formed mostly of cardiac muscle. The rest is formed of connective tissue fibers that form a dense network called the cardiac skeleton, giving structural support and shielding the electrical activity.

The endocardium is a white film of endothelium that lies on some additional connective tissue, and this lines the heart chambers. Speaking of chambers, the heart has four of them. These are the two atria and the two ventricles we talked about. The atria are separated by the intra-atrial septum, and the ventricles are separated by the interventricular septum.

The atria are the reception chambers where blood comes, which is subsequently pushed down into the ventricles. Oxygen-poor blood enters the right atrium by three different veins: the superior vena cava provides blood from upper areas of the body, the inferior vena cava delivers blood from lower portions of the body, and the coronary sinus collects blood draining from the myocardial. For the left atrium, there are four entryways, and these are the pulmonary veins, which bring blood from the lungs back to the heart.

The ventricles make up far more of the volume of the heart, and these are the actual circulation. The right ventricle sends blood into the pulmonary trunk, which flows to the lungs, while the left ventricle sends blood into the aorta, which is an artery, the largest one in the body. Another key characteristic is the heart valve, they ensure the unidirectional flow of blood, meaning they keep the blood traveling in the correct direction. There are two atrioventricular valves, or A valves, which connect each atrium to its corresponding ventricle. The right one is called the tricuspid valve, meaning it has three small flaps, and the left one is called the mitral or bicuspid valve, meaning it has two flaps. When the heart is relaxed, blood flows through, but when a ventricle contracts, the valve will close owing to the shift in pressure. There are two more valves called semilunar valves, and these are the aortic valve and the pulmonary valve.

These connect the ventricles and the arteries that arise from them, preventing blood that is exiting from going back into the ventricle. Now, let's dive a little deeper.

The heart has its very own varieties of muscle type: cardiac muscle, which is not found anywhere else in the body. Cardiac muscle fibers are comparable to skeletal muscle fibers in that they are striated, and the process of contraction with the sliding filaments is the same.

However, cardiac muscle fibers are not lengthy and multinucleated. Instead, they are short and plump, each with one or two nuclei, and they are branching and intertwined with one another.

The junctions connecting the cells are termed intercalated disks, and these contain desmosomes, which keep things together, and gap junctions, which allow for ions to move through.

The sarcomeres look similar to those found in skeletal muscle fibers, but there is more diversity in the diameters of the myofibrils, and there is more branching among them. Furthermore, the T-tubules enter each sarcomere twice, and the sarcoplasmic reticulum is somewhat simpler.

The method by which the heart pumps is comparable to what we already know about skeletal muscle cells in the action potential, but there are several major differences.

First, a small number of heart muscle cells can excite themselves; they do not need a nerve impulse. This is termed automaticity.

Also, contraction is extremely coordinated; all the fibers in the heart contract as a unit, and this is due to the gap junctions that tie everything together, allowing ions, consequently, depolarization to flow throughout the heart one cell at a time. Lastly, the refractory period is substantially longer in the heart, necessitating more time before another contraction can occur, which ensures the heart functions properly. One of the most fascinating aspects of the heart is its intrinsic cardiac conduction system.

There are certain specialized cells whose duty is not to contract but rather to distribute impulses throughout the heart to trigger contraction from within and also to guarantee that contraction is flawlessly coordinated.

These are called pacemaker cells, and they have an unstable resting potential that constantly depolarizes until the threshold is achieved. Problems with this mechanism are what contribute to arrhythmias and fibrillation, which are irregular heartbeats or fast contractions.

The heart also includes coronary arteries and coronary veins because the heart needs to be supplied with blood, just like any other organ.

CHAPTER TWO

Heart disease (Heart attack)

Healthy heart, so if you're wondering why heart disease is the leading cause of death, the answer is that people with chronic stress exist in our world, and chronic stress leads to the development of harmful daily routines. The harmful behaviors I refer to include, but are not limited to, inadequate sleep, a poor diet, and using unhealthy coping mechanisms like smoking as a way to manage stress. All of these actions put you at risk for heart disease risk factors, like excessive blood pressure, elevated cholesterol, becoming overweight, and getting diabetes.

There are items that can increase your chance of heart disease, such as risk letters. Your likelihood of developing heart disease increases with the number of risk factors you have. While certain risk factors, like your age, ethnic background, or family history, are unavoidable, the good news is that there are lots of things you can do to lower your risk.

Creating little and manageable changes to your daily routine can have a significant impact on your heart health and, in the long run, may save your life.

As of right now, the scientific term for this problem is heart disease, which refers to an illness of the blood veins that supply your heart with blood. The coronary arteries serve as the heart's own blood supply.

The heart is primarily composed of muscle. Because it guarantees that your heart can pump blood to the rest of your body efficiently, this blood supply is crucial. Plaque, a fatty substance, can accumulate inside your coronary arteries over time. Your arteries gradually narrow to the point where they are unable to supply your heart with adequate oxygen-rich blood due to a condition known as atherosclerosis.

A blood clot may form if a piece of plaque breaks off; this clot has the potential to obstruct your coronary artery and stop the flow of blood and oxygen to your heart muscle. We call this a heart attack. At the moment, heart disease progresses gradually over time and presents with a variety of symptoms.

Given that many of these risk factors hasten the process of atherosclerosis and that some people are unaware they have coronary heart disease until they experience a heart attack, it is imperative that you understand the risks and take steps to manage them in your life.

Let's start with stress, which is what I believe to be the root of a lot of these issues. The sensation of being overburdened or under strain is known as stress. Everyone has experienced it. It's possible that you're experiencing anxiety and panic. Perhaps you feel that you are being asked to do too much by others and that there aren't enough hours in the day. All right, that's a bit too much at this time.

That's normal to feel that way occasionally, and stress is necessary to accomplish goals, so it's not always a terrible thing. However, if you find it difficult to cope with these feelings over time, it's time to make some changes.

It's also vital to keep in mind that stress does not cause heart disease on its own. It's crucial to keep in mind that stress is not the cause of heart disease on its own; rather, stress is associated with bad behaviors that over time may raise your risk.

Stress increases the likelihood of developing bad habits such as smoking, overindulging in alcohol, and eating comfort food that is frequently heavy in fat or sugar.
While engaging in these activities can help us unwind, doing so too frequently over time can have negative effects on our health. While a brief rise in blood pressure is common when under stress, prolonged hypertension can result from stress-related

behaviors such as binge eating, excessive salt intake, excessive alcohol consumption, and insufficient physical activity. This can harm your arteries, heart, and other important organs. Over time, one in four people worldwide suffer from excessive blood pressure, and the majority of them are unaware of their own habits. Naturally, the mere pressure of time makes eating fast food more likely when you're anxious.

High cholesterol can result from consuming an excessive amount of meals high in saturated fat.
Your body contains cholesterol, a fatty material that has the ability to adhere to the artery walls.

It raises your risk of suffering a heart attack if it clogs or destroys the arteries.

Stress can lead to elevated blood pressure and cholesterol, and that eating an unbalanced diet and getting insufficient exercise can raise your risk of type 2 diabetes. Diabetes is a disorder in which the body is unable to regulate blood sugar levels due to either insufficient production of the hormone insulin or impaired insulin uptake.

I hope you're detecting a pattern here: it destroys your arteries, the blood vessels that deliver blood to your organs, putting your heart health at risk.

Your arteries are harmed if the builder consumes too much glucose or sugar in the blood. It is easier for fatty deposits to accumulate as a result of this artery injury. A heart attack may result from clogged and damaged arteries that provide blood to the heart.

Stress can be detrimental to your health when it becomes chronic or continues. Studies on the impact of stress on heart health have been ongoing for a while, especially since our stress response heavily involves the cardiovascular system.

An elevated risk of cardiovascular disease and coronary heart disease was linked to high levels of stress.
Furthermore, cardiomyopathy—a degenerative condition that weakens the heart muscle—may be predisposed to stress.

Research on the relationship between psychological well-being and heart health has demonstrated that the accumulation of daily stressors and major life events can both raise the risk of cardiovascular disease. Among them were:
Perceived stress. The amount of stress you feel you are experiencing right now is known as perceived stress.

Irrespective of the source, high levels of perceived stress have been associated with coronary heart disease and mortality related to coronary heart disease. Work-related stress. A 40 percent increase in the risk of cardiovascular disease has been linked to workplace or work-related stress.

Social seclusion. Loneliness and social isolation have been associated with a 50% higher chance of cardiovascular events such as a heart attack or stroke, as well as an increased risk of cardiovascular illness. Stress in early life.

Childhood stress or trauma has been associated with increased inflammatory markers and an increased chance of developing heart disease in later life.

A possible system?

Researchers have managed to establish a connection between cardiovascular disease and activity in the amygdala, a region of the brain. The processing of emotions like stress and terror is done by the amygdala. It contributes to the onset of the stress response as well.

Researchers discovered that increased production of white blood cells in the bone marrow was linked to increased activity in the amygdala, which in turn contributed to artery inflammation.

An increased risk of cardiovascular events such as angina (chest discomfort), heart attack, and stroke was also linked to increases in bone marrow activity and arterial inflammation. A smaller subset of patients who had both a brain scan and a psychological study showed that increased perceived stress was linked to increases in:
Behavior within the amygdala
Arterial inflammation and
C-reactive protein levels, which indicate the degree of inflammation in the body.

Since stress increases activity in the amygdala region of the brain, there is a connection between stress and heart disease.

This discovery has been connected to an increase in inflammation that is detrimental to the arteries. The chance of cardiovascular disease and other potentially dangerous occurrences seems to be increased by these alterations.
Other risk factors are also elevated by stress.
Diabetes and high blood pressure have also been associated with high stress levels.
Your risk of heart disease can be increased by either of these disorders.

Sleep is another risk factor that I find individuals overlook when it comes to their hearts. Your heart suffers when you get inadequate sleep.

In what ways does inadequate sleep negatively impact your heart? In conclusion, adults require seven hours of sleep on average.
Consider it analogous to recharging the body to guarantee optimal performance.

In addition to making you feel horrible, not getting enough sleep increases your risk of making poor decisions, including all the ones we've discussed. Now that we've covered all the negative aspects, let's discuss our next course of action.

I believe that I have all the researchers in a panic because listening to this will only cause your blood pressure to rise, which is something we really don't want.

The first thing to do is consider making gradual, small, healthy changes, such as consuming a day's worth of fiber or taking a quick stroll to relieve stress. Now is always the greatest time to make changes, no matter how minor. Though it's easy to put things off until later, you must act immediately if anything is negatively impacting your health. If you're not giving your all, you're not giving your family, friends, and coworkers the best either; thus, there will never be a perfect moment.

It's time to prioritize yourself, because doing so will prevent you from making decisions that raise your chance of developing heart disease.

Let's discuss the things you ought to stay away from. If you smoke, you ought to quit. It is the most crucial thing you can do for your overall well-being. It is bad for your health to smoke. I'll provide a link to it below. Try not to overindulge in alcohol— more than eight units for males and six for women in a single session. Not only can drinking have a detrimental effect on your liver and general health, but it also increases blood pressure, changes cholesterol, and causes weight gain.

The heart and sleep have a complex relationship. One layer is sleep quantity; individuals who don't get enough sleep are unable to supply their bodies with the necessary quantity of each stage of sleep for optimal functioning.

The quality of sleep is also crucial.
Even if you get adequate sleep, it might occasionally be shallow and sporadic, which keeps your body from getting the maintenance it needs during that period of time. Other dimensions are also significant. In addition to improving blood pressure, blood sugar, and weight management, getting adequate sleep is beneficial for heart health.

Consistently getting enough sleep is also beneficial for controlling blood pressure, blood sugar, and weight. As heart disorders like heart attacks and strokes are linked to these health issues, controlling these risk factors and obtaining enough sleep can be very beneficial.

As a result of insomnia, sleep loss stresses the body and releases cortisol, which may hasten atherosclerosis.

Let's now discuss food. Eat a healthy, balanced diet that includes lots of fruits and vegetables. Of course, you can indulge yourself occasionally, but if that starts to happen every day, you may need to make some changes.

Also, take advantage of every opportunity to get up and move. Engaging in regular physical activity lowers your chance of heart disease. Being more physically active can reduce your risk of heart disease by 35%. If the thought of engaging in any physical activity makes you feel anxious or as though you don't have enough time, start small.

Finding the time to engage in physical activity can be challenging, but if you incorporate it into activities you already do, you'll be much more likely to form a habit you want to stick with.

Examples of such activities include walking to work instead of driving, getting off the bus a few stops early, or using the stairs instead of the elevator. Make a list of everything you do each day, and see when you can find 10 minutes or more to engage in physical activity. Small actions add up to have significant effects.

General causes of heart disease (hidden and deadly)

Many factors can lead to heart disease, some of which are potentially fatal and obscure. It is noteworthy that heart disorders frequently have several contributing causes, indicating that multiple factors may play a role in their development. The following are some typical reasons, some of which may be fatal and/or concealed:

1. **Poor Diet**: Unknown Factor: Heart disease can be caused by consuming too many processed foods, large amounts of saturated and trans fats, and too much salt.

• Processed Foods: Processed foods frequently contain large amounts of added sugars, processed carbs, and harmful fats. Usually, when these foods are processed, important nutrients and fiber are removed, and artificial additives and preservatives are added.

Effect on Heart Health: Research has connected regular consumption of processed foods to inflammation, weight gain, and insulin resistance. These elements play a role in the emergence of diseases, including type 2 diabetes and obesity, which increase the risk of heart disease.

•Saturated and Trans Fats: While trans fats are frequently found in partly hydrogenated oils used in many processed and fried meals, saturated fats are typically found in animal products like red meat, full-fat dairy, and tropical oils.

Effect on Heart Health: Low-density lipoprotein, or LDL, cholesterol is sometimes referred to as "bad" cholesterol. Saturated and trans fats can both raise LDL cholesterol levels. Increased risk of heart attacks and strokes as well as atherosclerosis are caused by the buildup of atherosclerotic plaques in arteries, which are facilitated by elevated low-density lipoprotein (LDL) cholesterol.

• Overconsumption of salt: The body needs sodium, a mineral found in salt.

However, consuming too much sodium— often the result of a diet heavy in salt—can have negative health effects.

Effect on Cardiovascular Health: An increased risk of hypertension (high blood pressure) is linked to a high-salt diet. The increased effort required by hypertension on the heart to pump blood results in arterial strain and a higher risk of heart-related conditions, such as heart attacks and heart failure.

2. **Physical Inactivity**: A Hidden Factor Desk employment and sedentary lifestyles can have a role in the development of cardiac illnesses. A lack of consistent exercise or physical activity is referred to as physical inactivity.

It includes leading a lifestyle with little exercise and little participation in activities that increase heart rate and enhance general fitness.

Effect on Cardiovascular Health: It is essential to engage in regular physical activity to preserve cardiovascular health. Being physically inactive can cause a number of health problems, such as an elevated risk of heart disease.

• Sedentary Lifestyles: Sedentary lifestyles involve little to no physical activity and long stretches of sitting or lying down. This relates to a number of facets of daily life, such as employment, recreation, and travel.

Effect on Cardiovascular Health: Decreased Level of Physical Fitness Reduced cardiovascular fitness from inactivity can affect how well the heart and lungs function to pump oxygen and nutrients throughout the body.

• Desk Jobs: A lot of modern jobs, particularly those involving desk work, require employees to sit for extended periods of time.

This sedentary lifestyle can be a major factor in the general lack of physical activity.

Effect on Cardiovascular Health:

Muscle Inactivity: Extended sitting can cause a lack of movement in the muscles, especially the lower back and legs.

The body's capacity to effectively use glucose and control insulin is diminished by this lack of muscular action.

Impaired Blood Circulation: Extended periods of sitting can impair blood circulation, which raises the risk of blood clots and causes blood to pool in the legs.

Deep vein thrombosis (DVT) and, consequently, cardiovascular problems may be exacerbated by this.

• Psychological Impact: Engaging in physical activity is good for one's body and mind. Sedentary habits have an indirect negative impact on heart health because they can exacerbate stress, anxiety, and despair.

Effect on Cardiovascular Health:
Heart issues brought on by stress: Chronic stress, which is frequently linked to sedentary lifestyles, can affect blood pressure, heart rate, and inflammation, all of which can lead to the development of cardiac disorders.

Intervention and Prevention:
Regular exercise and a change in lifestyle can help to lessen the detrimental effects of physical inactivity on heart health.

Exercise Prescription: Regular aerobic, strength, and flexibility workouts help control weight, enhance cardiovascular health, and lower the risk of heart disease.

Active Lifestyle Promotion: Incorporating physical exercise into everyday routines, such as walking, taking stairs, or taking breaks from lengthy sitting, can have a favorable effect on heart health.

Public health initiatives: To promote physical activity and lower the incidence of sedentary lifestyles, community-based programs, corporate wellness initiatives and educational campaigns are essential.

In conclusion, physical inactivity can hasten the onset of heart disease through a variety of physiological and metabolic pathways, particularly when combined with sedentary lifestyles linked to desk occupations or a lack of exercise. Regular physical exercise promotion is crucial for preserving cardiovascular health and lowering the risk of heart-related problems.

3. **Genetics**: Hidden Factor: Even if other lifestyle factors appear normal, an individual's risk may be increased by a family history of heart disease.
The risk of heart disease in an individual is mostly determined by their genetic makeup.

The form and functionality of the heart, blood vessels, and other cardiovascular system components can be influenced by specific genetic variables.

Certain genetic mutations or changes may be inherited by some people, predisposing them to illnesses such as hypertension, excessive cholesterol, or specific cardiac problems.

Heart disease is known to "cluster" in families, which means that those who have close relatives (parents, siblings) with the same disease may be more likely to get a heart disease themselves.

Hidden element: People may carry genetic predispositions without exhibiting obvious symptoms or indicators, which is the hidden element in genetics and cardiac disorders.

This implies that a person's genetic composition may still affect their propensity to heart disease even if they lead an apparently healthy lifestyle.

Silent Progression: Without obvious or immediate symptoms, genetic factors may have a silent role in the silent development of cardiovascular problems. People need to be conscious of their genetic predispositions and family history because of this.

Typical genetic contributors:
Genetic Variations and Cholesterol Metabolism: Genetic variations can impact the body's cholesterol metabolism.

Atherosclerosis risk may increase in certain people due to a genetic predisposition to increased LDL (low-density lipoprotein) cholesterol levels.

Blood Pressure Regulation: The regulation of blood pressure can be influenced by genetic factors. People who have a family history of high blood pressure may be more likely to experience high blood pressure themselves.

cardiac rhythm disorders: Individuals may be predisposed to structural cardiac abnormalities or irregular heart rhythms (arrhythmias) by specific genetic mutations.

Interaction with Lifestyle Factors: Modifiable Risk Factors: People who have a family history of heart disease should be especially mindful of their diet, level of activity, and tobacco use.

Choosing a healthy lifestyle can help reduce the hazards associated with genetics.

Personalized Prevention: More individualized preventive and intervention techniques are possible when one is aware of their genetic predispositions. For people with a family history of heart disease, routine health examinations and tests may be advised.

Polygenic Risk: Heart disorders are frequently polygenic, which means that a number of different genetic variants work together to cause them.

Cumulative Influence: An individual's total risk profile is influenced by a combination of environmental factors and various genetic variants. Because of this intricacy, using genetics alone to predict and prevent cardiac problems is difficult.

Genetic Testing: Thanks to developments in the field, people can now determine their genetic susceptibility to a number of illnesses, such as heart disorders.
Early Detection: Certain genetic markers linked to an elevated risk of heart disease can be found through genetic testing. In order to lower the risk, early detection enables proactive management and lifestyle changes.

Implications for Public Health: Understanding the role of genetics in cardiac disorders has consequences for public health.
Screening Programs: Targeted screening programs for people with a family history of heart disease may be part of public health initiatives.

Early risk factor identification can result in better management and preventative plans. In conclusion, a person's genetic makeup can greatly influence their chance of acquiring heart disease. Even when lifestyle factors seem normal, a family history of heart disease acts as a hidden factor that affects the risk.

In order to manage and lower the risk of heart disease in those with a family history, it can be crucial to recognize one's genetic predispositions, adopt a heart-healthy lifestyle, and seek early medical attention.

4. **Psychosocial Factors**: Hidden Factor: Prolonged stress, melancholy, and social isolation might affect heart health and play a role in the onset of cardiac conditions. The psychological and social components that affect a person's entire social environment and mental health are referred to as psychosocial factors.

Three important psychosocial factors that can have a significant impact on heart health are social isolation, depression, and chronic stress.

Effect on Cardiovascular Health: Biological Reactions: The body may experience biological reactions as a result of these psychosocial factors.

These reactions may include the sympathetic nervous system being activated and the release of stress hormones like cortisol, which may eventually have an effect on the cardiovascular system.

Chronic Stress: Characterized by a protracted condition of both physiological and psychological strain, chronic stress is frequently brought on by continuous obstacles in life, pressures at work, or personal struggles.

Repercussions

Elevated Blood Pressure: Extended periods of stress can raise blood pressure, which puts stress on the heart and raises the possibility of hypertension, a significant risk factor for heart disease.

Inflammation: Prolonged stress triggers the body's inflammatory response, which in turn fuels atherosclerosis and other cardiovascular problems.

• Depression: This mood illness is defined by enduring melancholy, hopelessness, and disinterest in or enjoyment from activities.

Effect on Cardiovascular Health:

Changes in Heart Rate Variability: Heart rate variability is a measure of cardiovascular health and has been associated with depression.

Adverse cardiovascular events are linked to a higher likelihood of reduced heart rate variability.

Inflammatory Pathways: Pro-inflammatory conditions that affect the cardiovascular system are exacerbated by depression, which is also linked to elevated blood levels of inflammatory markers.

•Social Isolation: The absence of social ties, relationships, and a feeling of belonging is referred to as social isolation.

Effect on Cardiovascular Health:

Stress and Loneliness: Chronic stress and feelings of loneliness are two outcomes of social isolation that are detrimental to heart.

Better Health Practices: On the other hand, social ties can have a beneficial impact on better health practices. Strong social support networks increase an individual's likelihood of participating in heart-healthy activities like regular exercise and eating a balanced diet.

Psychosocial therapies: Including psychosocial therapies can improve mental health and, in turn, heart health. These interventions include stress reduction methods, counseling, and support groups. Integrated treatment: For complete cardiovascular treatment, an integrated strategy that takes into account factors related to both physical and mental health is necessary.

In conclusion, there are a number of unspoken variables that can have a substantial negative influence on heart health and hasten the onset of heart illnesses, including chronic stress, despair, and social isolation.

It is essential to identify and treat these psychological factors with interventions, support networks, and holistic methods in order to enhance general health and lower the risk of cardiovascular problems.

CHAPTER THREE

You are having a heart attack – What should you do?

Knowing what to do as soon as you suspect a heart attack and being able to identify its symptoms can literally save lives. When blood supply to a portion of the heart muscle is interrupted, usually by a blood clot, the result is a heart attack, also known as a myocardial infarction. In these kinds of situations, time is of the essence, and knowing what steps to take right away can help minimize harm and improve the likelihood of a full recovery.

We'll talk about what to do in this session if you think you could be having a heart attack and stress the need for prompt action and having access to emergency medical care. Make an emergency help request.

One of the most important things to do when experiencing a heart attack is to call for emergency assistance. This will guarantee that qualified medical help will arrive quickly and can offer specialist care. This is a detailed guide explaining how to contact for emergency help:

1. **Identify the signs and symptoms**: It's critical to identify the warning signs and symptoms of a heart attack prior to dialing 911.

In addition to pain or discomfort in the arms, back, neck, jaw, or stomach, these symptoms might also include nausea, lightheadedness, shortness of breath, and chest pain or discomfort.

2. **Don't Hesitate**: In the event of a heart attack, timing is vital. The possible damage to the heart muscle increases with the length of time that passes before seeking medical attention. It's critical to take immediate action and to recognize how terrible the situation is.

3. **Make an Emergency Services Call**: The emergency services number is 911, although it may differ in many other countries.

It is imperative to be aware of the emergency number in your area and to call it right away if you think someone is having a heart attack.

If you are having the symptoms and you are with someone else in a public location, ask them to call.

4. **Provide Necessary Information**:
Remain composed and provide pertinent information when speaking with the emergency dispatcher. Declare unequivocally that you believe you are having a heart attack, and list the symptoms you are experiencing.

Provide emergency responders with a precise location, including any cross streets or landmarks, so they can get to you faster.

5. **Comply with dispatcher guidelines**: While awaiting the arrival of assistance, the dispatcher could offer instructions. Pay close attention to their instructions.

They may ask you to do particular things, like staying on the line, taking prescribed drugs (like aspirin), or giving them details about the circumstances.

6. **Remain with the Individual**: If you are with someone who is having a heart attack, stay by their side until assistance comes. Reassure the person and make an effort to keep them composed.

Cardiopulmonary resuscitation (CPR) may be administered by the dispatcher until emergency medical assistance comes if they lose consciousness and cease breathing properly.

7. Get Ready for Emergency Medical Services (EMS) to Arrive:

Prepare to direct emergency personnel to the site, particularly if it is not easily accessible. Tell the dispatcher if there are any barriers or special instructions to contact the person who is in distress.

Recall that the first and most important step in surviving a heart attack is to contact someone for immediate assistance.

Prompt action can decrease long-term heart damage and greatly increase the likelihood of a favorable outcome.
Each country has different emergency contact numbers, so when you travel to a new area, it's critical to know what the local emergency services are.

These are a few widely used emergency phone numbers across different nations:
USA: 911
Canada: 911
England and Wales: 999 or 112.
European Union: 112
Australia: 000
New Zealand: 111

India: 101 (fire), 102 (ambulance), and 100 (police).

Police in South Africa: 10111; ambulance: 10177

China: 120 (ambulance), 110 (police)

Japan: 119 (fire/ambulance), 110 (police).

Korea, South: 112

Brazil: 192 (ambulance), 190 (police).

Mexico: 911

Russia: 112

First Aid Methods

The term "positioning the victim" describes how to best situate and arrange a person who might be in distress or experiencing a medical emergency so as to limit potential harm and increase their well-being.

This is frequently an essential component of emergency response and first aid.

A guide for helping the victim sit down and keep calm:

Sitting down: In certain cases, having the victim sit down can help prevent falls and injuries. It also allows individuals to preserve energy and avoid unnecessary stress on their bodies.

Remaining calm: Encouraging the victim to be calm is vital for their mental well-being and can even have favorable impacts on their physical state. Panic and anxiety can exacerbate certain medical issues, so keeping a sense of calm might be useful.

The importance of avoiding needless physical exertion:

Energy conservation: Excessive physical exertion during a medical emergency or other distress situation can be harmful to the victim's health. Energy conservation is essential, particularly for conditions that could be made worse by physical exertion. Keeping things from getting worse: Excessive movement or physical activity can make wounds or illnesses worse.

For instance, difficulties may arise from severe physical exertion in cases of trauma or specific cardiovascular conditions. In conclusion, encouraging someone who appears to be in distress to sit down and maintain composure can improve that person's general wellbeing.

Furthermore, it's critical to refrain from needless physical exertion in order to stop additional damage and enable the person to preserve energy—especially during an emergency. When offering aid, keep the particulars and nature of the medical issue in mind at all times. It is essential to seek professional medical assistance if the condition is serious.

CHAPTER FOUR

Reversing heart attack for life

Reversing the damage caused by a heart attack is a difficult procedure that often involves medical intervention and lifestyle adjustments. Here are some general tips that may contribute to heart health Medical Treatment: Prompt medical care is crucial during a heart attack. Treatment may involve drugs, procedures like angioplasty or stent implantation, or, in severe circumstances, coronary artery bypass surgery.

Following the prescribed medications, such as antiplatelet meds, beta-blockers, and statins, can assist regulate heart health.

Cardiac Rehabilitation: Cardiac rehabilitation programs, supervised by healthcare specialists, can assist in the recovery process. These programs frequently incorporate exercise, instruction on heart-healthy lifestyle, and emotional support.

Lifestyle Changes: Adopting a heart-healthy diet, which often means consuming more fruits, vegetables, whole grains, lean proteins, and minimizing saturated fats, trans fats, cholesterol, and sodium.

Regular physical activity is vital. Consult with healthcare providers to establish an exercise regimen fit for your condition.

Quitting smoking is vital, as smoking is a significant risk factor for heart disease.

Managing stress with relaxation techniques, meditation, or counseling may also be effective.

Monitoring and Managing Risk Factors: Regular monitoring of blood pressure, cholesterol levels, and blood sugar can assist manage cardiovascular risk factors.

Weight management is vital, as obesity can lead to heart disease.

It's crucial to highlight that the capacity to "reverse" the damage produced by a heart attack depends on numerous circumstances, including the level of damage, the timeliness of medical intervention, and the individual's overall health.

Always speak with healthcare specialists for specialized advice and assistance based on your individual situation. They can provide information specific to your health situation and assist you on the most appropriate course of action.

CHAPTER FIVE

The easy heart cure food list

Embracing a heart-healthy lifestyle entails thoughtful eating choices. "The Simple Heart Cure Food List" is a curated list of healthy foods known for supporting cardiovascular well-being. By including these easy yet powerful choices into your diet, you hope to enhance heart health and lower the risk of cardiovascular diseases. Always contact with healthcare professionals for individualized guidance on maintaining a healthy heart.

Fruits and vegetables:

Berries

Leafy greens

Citrus fruits

Apples

Avocados

Broccoli

Carrots

Whole Grains:

Oats

Brown rice

Quinoa

Whole wheat

Barley

Lean Proteins:

Fatty fish (salmon, mackerel, and trout)

Skinless poultry

Legumes (beans, lentils)

Tofu

Nuts and seeds (moderation)

Healthy Fats:

Olive oil

Canola oil

Nuts and seeds

Avocados

Dairy:

low in fat or fat-free (milk, yogurt, cheese)

Lean Meats:

Lean slices of beef or pork

Herbs and Spices: Garlic

Turmeric

Ginger

Cinnamon Beverages:

Water, green tea

Moderate amounts of coffee (without extra-added sweeteners or cream)

Limit or avoid:

Processed and red meats

Trans fats and partly hydrogenated oils

Excessive salt/sodium

Added sugars and sugary beverages

This list covers full, nutrient-dense foods that are generally acknowledged as healthy for heart health. Always speak with a healthcare expert for individualized advice based on your specific health condition.

CONCLUSION

In conclusion, "Heart Disease (Heart Attack): Guide to a Healthy Heart" functions as an all-encompassing travel guide for persons who are interested in putting their cardiovascular health at the forefront of their priorities. Readers have learned essential knowledge about the complexities of heart health as a result of their journey through the pages of this enlightening guide, which has enabled them to make lifestyle decisions that are informed by the information they acquired.

As we get to the end of this chapter, let us not forget that a healthy heart is not only the result of advances in medical technology, but also, and this is the most essential point, the consequence of the choices we make on a daily basis in order to take care of our health. We hope that this guide will motivate you to make a commitment to living a lifestyle that is heart-conscious, so creating long-term health and vitality for all those who embark on the journey to a heart that is stronger and happier.

Heart Disease (Heart Attack)

www.ingramcontent.com/pod-product-compliance
Lightning Source LLC
Chambersburg PA
CBHW071100290526
45795CB00004B/1580